Air Fryer Cookb

Your Lunch & Dinner

Easy & Healthy Recipes to Make

Unforgettable First Courses

Eva Sheppard

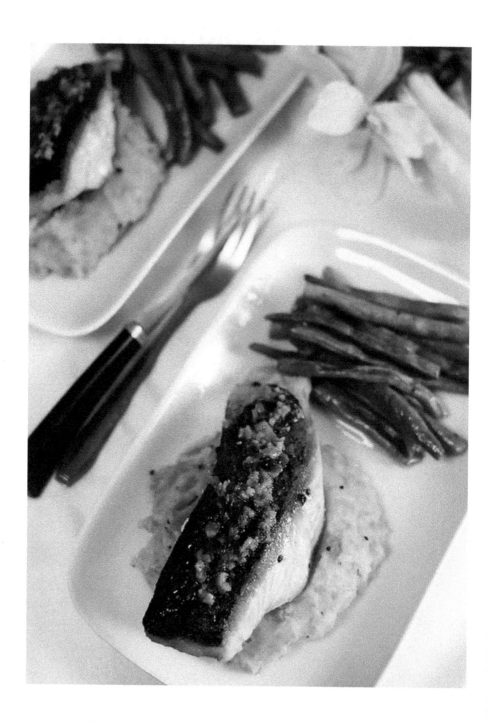

© **Copyright 2021 - All rights reserved.**

The content contained within this book may not be reproduced, duplicated or transmitted without direct written permission from the author or the publisher. Under no circumstances will any blame or legal responsibility be held against the publisher, or author, for any damages, reparation, or monetary loss due to the information contained within this book. Either directly or indirectly.

Legal Notice:

This book is copyright protected. This book is only for personal use. You cannot amend, distribute, sell, use, quote or paraphrase any part, or the content within this book, without the consent of the author or publisher.

Disclaimer Notice:

Please note the information contained within this document is for educational and entertainment purposes only. All effort has been executed to present accurate, up to date, and reliable, complete information. No warranties of any kind are declared or implied. Readers acknowledge that the author is not engaging in the rendering of legal, financial, medical or professional advice. The content within this book has been derived from various sources. Please consult a licensed professional before attempting any techniques outlined in this book.

By reading this document, the reader agrees that under no circumstances is the author responsible for any losses, direct or indirect, which are incurred as a result of the use of information contained within this document, including, but not limited to, — errors, omissions, or inaccuracies.

TABLE OF CONTENT

Pantano Romanesco with Goat Cheese Appetizer

Preparation Time: 20 minutes

Servings 4

Nutrition Values: 237 Calories; 20.4g Fat; 0.9g Carbs; 13g Protein; 0.9g Sugars

Ingredients

- 6 ounces goat cheese, sliced
- 2 shallots, thinly sliced
- 2 Pantano Romanesco tomatoes, cut into 1/2-inch slices
- 1 ½ tablespoons extra-virgin olive oil
- 3/4 teaspoon sea salt
- Fresh parsley, for garnish
- Fresh basil, chopped

Directions

1. Preheat your air fryer to 380 degrees F.

2. Now, pat each tomato slice dry using a paper towel. Sprinkle each slice with salt

8

and chopped basil. Top with a slice of goat cheese.

3. Top with the shallot slices; drizzle with olive oil. Add the prepared tomato and feta "bites" to the air fryer food basket.

4. Cook in the air fryer for about 14 minutes. Lastly, adjust seasonings to taste and serve garnished with fresh parsley leaves. Enjoy!

Swiss Chard and Cheese Omelet

Preparation Time: 25 minutes

Servings 2

Nutrition Values: 388 Calories; 27g Fat; 6g Carbs; 29g Protein; 2.6g Sugars

Ingredients

- 1 teaspoon garlic paste
- 1 ½ tablespoons olive oil
- 1/2 cup crème fraîche
- 1/3 teaspoon ground black pepper, to your liking
- 1/3 cup Swiss cheese, crumbled
- 1 teaspoon cayenne pepper
- 1/3 cup Swiss chard, torn into pieces
- 5 eggs
- 1/4 cup yellow onions, chopped
- 1 teaspoon fine sea salt

Directions

1. Crack your eggs into a mixing dish; then, add the crème fraîche, salt, ground black pepper, and cayenne pepper.

2. Next, coat the inside of a baking dish with olive oil and tilt it to spread evenly. Scrape the egg/cream mixture into the baking dish. Add the other ingredients; mix to combine well.

3. Bake for 18 minutes at 292 degrees F. Serve immediately.

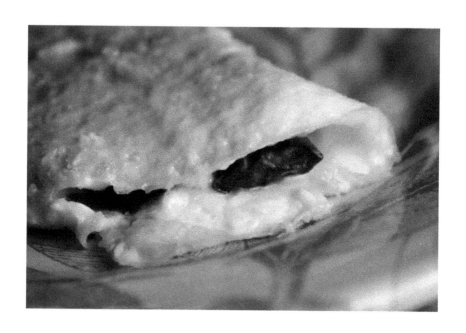

Mom's Jacket Potatoes

Preparation Time: 23 minutes

Servings 4

Nutrition Values: 270 Calories; 10.9g Fat; 35.2g Carbs; 8.8g Protein; 2.8g Sugars

Ingredients

- 1/3 cup Cottage cheese, softened
- 1/3 cup Parmigiano-Reggiano cheese, grated
- 1 teaspoon black pepper
- 1 ½ heaping tablespoons roughly chopped cilantro leaves
- 1/3 cup green onions, finely chopped
- 5 average-sized potatoes
- 2 ½ tablespoons softened butter
- 1 teaspoon salt

Directions

1. Firstly, stab your potatoes with a fork. Cook them in the air fryer basket for 20 minutes at 345 degrees F.

2. While the potatoes are cooking, make the filling by mixing the rest of the above ingredients.

3. Afterward, open the potatoes up and stuff them with the prepared filling. Bon appétit!

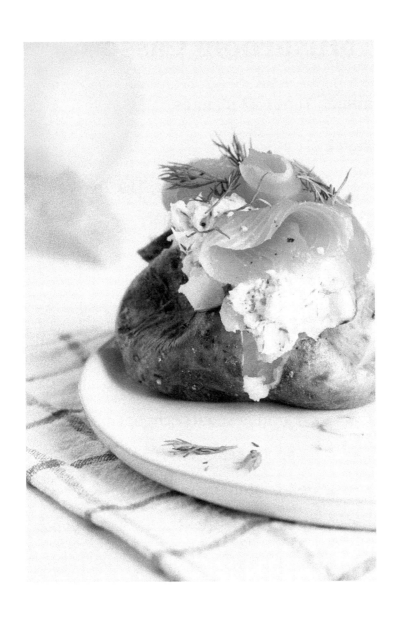

Skinny Asparagus and Mushroom Casserole

Preparation Time: 27 minutes

Servings 2

Nutrition Values: 207 Calories; 19.7g Fat; 30.2g Carbs; 20.6g Protein; 3.7g Sugars

Ingredients

- 1/3 cup milk
- 1/3 cup Colby cheese, grated
- 5 slices of Italian bread, cut into cubes
- 1 1/2 cups white mushrooms, sliced
- 2 asparagus spears, chopped
- 1 teaspoon table salt, or to taste
- 2 well-beaten eggs
- 1/3 teaspoon smoked cayenne pepper
- 1 teaspoon ground black pepper, or to taste
- 1/3 teaspoon dried rosemary, crushed

Directions

1. Throw the bread cubes into the baking dish.

2. In a mixing dish, thoroughly combine the eggs and milk. Stir in 1/2 of cheese; add the seasonings. Pour 3/4 of egg/cheese mixture over the bread cubes in the baking dish; press gently using a wide spatula.

3. Now, top with the mushrooms and chopped asparagus. Pour the remaining egg/cheese mixture over the top; make sure to spread it evenly.

Top with the remaining Colby cheese and bake for 20 minutes at 325 degrees F.

Winter Sausage with Root Vegetables

Preparation Time: 30 minutes

Servings 4

Nutrition Values:289 Calories; 13.6g Fat; 32.5g Carbs; 13.3g Protein; 6.7g Sugars

Ingredients

- 1/2 pound Italian sausage
- 3 sprigs rosemary
- 1 medium-sized parsnip, sliced
- 1/3 pound fingerling potatoes
- 3 sprigs thyme
- 1/3 pound carrots, trimmed and cut into matchsticks
- 1/2 celery stalk, sliced
- 2 garlic cloves, smashed
- 2 tablespoons extra-virgin olive oil
- 3 small-sized leeks, cut into halves lengthwise

- A pinch of grated nutmeg

- Salt and black pepper, to taste

Directions

1. Arrange fingerling potatoes, carrots, celery, parsnip, and leeks on the bottom of the air fryer baking dish. Tuck the garlic cloves around the vegetables.

2. Sprinkle with the seasonings and top with the sausage.

3. Roast approximately 33 minutes at 375 degrees F, stirring occasionally. Bon appétit!

Chinese Cod Fillets

Preparation time: 10 minutes

Cooking time: 15 minutes

Servings: 4

Ingredients:

- 4 cod fillets, boneless
- Salt and black pepper to taste
- 1 cup water
- 4 tablespoons light soy sauce
- 1 tablespoon sugar
- 3 tablespoons olive oil + a drizzle
- 4 ginger slices
- 3 spring onions, chopped
- 2 tablespoons coriander, chopped

Directions:

1. Season the fish with salt and pepper, then drizzle some oil over it and rub well.

2. Put the fish in your air fryer and cook at 360 degrees F for 12 minutes.

3. Put the water in a pot and heat up over medium heat; add the soy sauce and sugar, stir, bring to a simmer, and remove from the heat.

4. Heat up a pan with the olive oil over medium heat; add the ginger and green onions, stir, cook for 2-3 minutes, and remove from the heat.

5. Divide the fish between plates and top with ginger, coriander, and green onions.

6. Drizzle the soy sauce mixture all over, serve, and enjoy!

Nutrition Values: calories 270, fat 12, fiber 8, carbs 16, protein 14

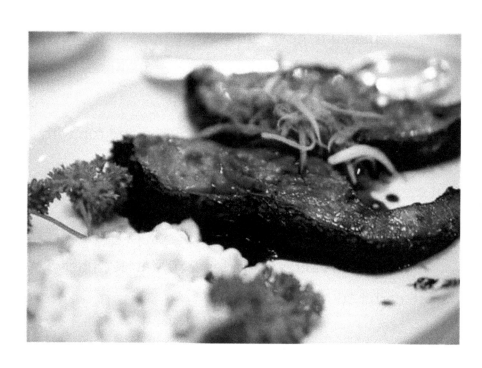

Cod Fillets with Leeks

Preparation time: 10 minutes

Cooking time: 15 minutes

Servings: 2

Ingredients:

- 2 black cod fillets, boneless
- 1 tablespoon olive oil
- Salt and black pepper to taste
- 2 leeks, sliced
- ½ cup pecans, chopped

Directions:

1. In a bowl, mix the cod with the oil, salt, pepper, and the leeks; toss / coat well.

2. Transfer the cod to your air fryer and cook at 360 degrees F for 15 minutes.

3. Divide the fish and leeks between plates, sprinkle the pecans on top, and serve immediately.

Nutrition Values: calories 280, fat 4, fiber 2, carbs 12, protein 15

Rosemary Shrimp Kabobs

Preparation time: 5 minutes

Cooking time: 7 minutes

Servings: 2

Ingredients:

- 8 shrimps, peeled and deveined
- 4 garlic cloves, minced
- Salt and black pepper to taste
- 8 red bell pepper slices
- 1 tablespoon rosemary, chopped
- 1 tablespoon olive oil

Directions:

1. Place all ingredients in a bowl and toss them well.

2. Thread 2 shrimp and 2 bell pepper slices on a skewer, and then repeat with 2 more shrimp and bell pepper slices.

3. Thred another 2 shrimp and 2 bell pepper slices on the other skewer and then repeat

with the last 2 shrimp and 2 bell pepper slices.

4. Put the kabobs in your air fryer's basket., cook at 360 degrees F for 7 minutes and serve immediately with a side salad.

Nutrition Values: calories 200, fat 4, fiber 12, carbs 15, protein 6

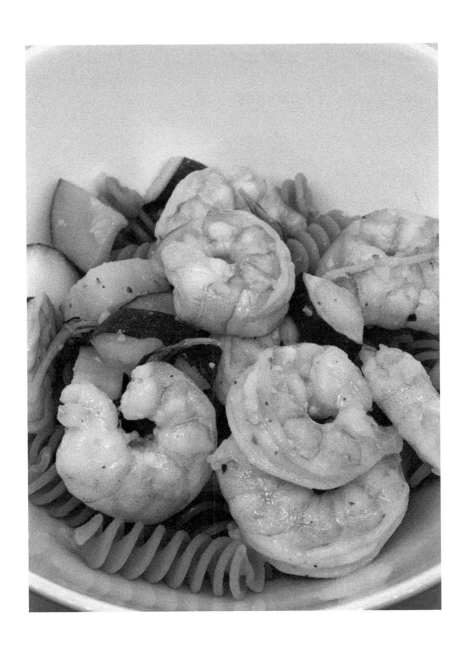

Simple Balsamic Cod Fillets

Preparation time: 5 minutes

Cooking time: 12 minutes

Servings: 2

Ingredients:

- 2 cod fillets, boneless
- 2 tablespoons lemon juice
- Salt and black pepper to taste
- ½ teaspoon garlic powder
- ⅓ cup water
- ⅓ cup balsamic vinegar
- 3 shallots, chopped
- 2 tablespoons olive oil

Directions:

1. In a bowl, toss the cod with the salt, pepper, lemon juice, garlic powder, water, vinegar, and oil; coat well.

2. Transfer the fish to your fryer's basket and cook at 360 degrees F for 12 minutes, flipping them halfway.

3. Divide the fish between plates, sprinkle the shallots on top, and serve.

Nutrition Values: calories 271, fat 12, fiber 10, carbs 16, protein 20

Chili Salmon Fillets

Preparation time: 5 minutes

Cooking time: 8 minutes

Servings: 2

Ingredients:

- 2 salmon fillets, boneless
- Salt and black pepper to taste
- 3 red chili peppers, chopped
- 2 tablespoons lemon juice
- 2 tablespoon olive oil
- 2 tablespoon garlic, minced

Directions:

1. In a bowl, combine the ingredients, toss, and coat fish well.

2. Transfer everything to your air fryer and cook at 365 degrees F for 8 minutes, flipping the fish halfway.

3. Divide between plates and serve right away.

Nutrition Values: c alories 280, fat 4, fiber 8, carbs 15, protein 20

Shrimp and Veggie Mix

Preparation time: 10 minutes

Cooking time: 20 minutes

Servings: 4

Ingredients:

- ½ cup red onion, chopped
- 1 cup red bell pepper, chopped
- 1 cup celery, chopped
- 1 pound shrimp, peeled and deveined
- 1 teaspoon Worcestershire sauce
- Salt and black pepper to taste
- 1 tablespoon butter, melted
- 1 teaspoon sweet paprika

Directions:

1. Add all the ingredients to a bowl and mix well.

2. Transfer everything to your air fryer and cook 320 degrees F for 20 minutes, shaking halfway.

3. Divide between plates and serve.

Nutrition Values: calories 220, fat 14, fiber 9, carbs 17, protein 20

White Fish and Peas

Preparation time: 10 minutes

Cooking time: 12 minutes

Servings: 4

Ingredients:

- 4 white fish fillets, boneless
- 2 tablespoons cilantro, chopped
- 2 cups peas, cooked and drained
- 4 tablespoons veggie stock
- ½ teaspoon basil, dried
- ½ teaspoon sweet paprika
- 2 garlic cloves, minced
- Salt and pepper to taste

Directions:

1. In a bowl, mix the fish with all ingredients except the peas; toss to coat the fish well.

2. Transfer everything to your air fryer and cook at 360 degrees F for 12 minutes.

3. Add the peas, toss, and divide everything between plates.

4. Serve and enjoy.

Nutrition Values: calories 241, fat 8, fiber 12, carbs 15, protein 18

Cod and Lime Sauce

Preparation time: 5 minutes

Cooking time: 12 minutes

Servings: 4

Ingredients:

- 4 cod fillets, boneless
- Salt and black pepper to taste
- 3 teaspoons lime zest
- 2 teaspoons lime juice
- 3 tablespoons chives, chopped
- 6 tablespoons butter, melted
- 2 tablespoons olive oil

Directions:

1. Season the fish with the salt and pepper, rub it with the oil, and then put it in your air fryer.

2. Cook at 360 degrees F for 10 minutes, flipping once.

3. Heat up a pan with the butter over medium heat, and then add the chives, salt, pepper, lime juice, and zest, whisk; cook for 1-2 minutes.

4. Divide the fish between plates, drizzle the lime sauce all over, and serve immediately.

Nutrition Values: calories 280, fat 12, fiber 9, carbs 17, protein 15

Flavored Salmon Fillets

Preparation time: 5 minutes

Cooking time: 12 minutes

Servings: 4

Ingredients:

- 4 salmon fillets, boneless
- 1 tablespoon olive oil
- Salt and black pepper to taste
- 1 teaspoon cumin, ground
- 1 teaspoon sweet paprika
- ½ teaspoon chili powder
- 1 teaspoon garlic powder
- Juice of 1 lime

Directions:

1. In a bowl, mix the salmon with the other ingredients, rub / coat well, and transfer to your air fryer.

2. Cook at 350 degrees F for 6 minutes on each side.

3. Divide the fish between plates and serve right away with a side salad.

Nutrition Values: calories 280, fat 14, fiber 4, carbs 18, protein 20

Tasty Air Fried Cod

Preparation time: 10 minutes

Cooking time: 12 minutes

Servings: 4

Ingredients:

- 2 cod fish, 7 ounces each
- A drizzle of sesame oil
- Salt and black pepper to the taste
- 1 cup water
- 1 teaspoon dark soy sauce
- 4 tablespoons light soy sauce
- 1 tablespoon sugar
- 3 tablespoons olive oil
- 4 ginger slices
- 3 spring onions, chopped
- 2 tablespoons coriander, chopped

Directions:

1. Season fish with salt, pepper, drizzle sesame oil, rub well and leave aside for 10 minutes.

2. Add fish to your air fryer and cook at 356 degrees F for 12 minutes.

3. Meanwhile, heat up a pot with the water over medium heat, add dark and light soy sauce and sugar, stir, bring to a simmer and take off heat.

4. Heat up a pan with the olive oil over medium heat, add ginger and green onions, stir, cook for a few minutes and take off heat.

5. Divide fish on plates, top with ginger and green onions, drizzle soy sauce mix, sprinkle coriander and serve right away.

6. Enjoy!

Nutrition Values: calories 300, fat 17, fiber 8, carbs 20, protein 22

Delicious Catfish

Preparation time: 10 minutes

Cooking time: 20 minutes

Servings: 4

Ingredients:

- 4 cat fish fillets
- Salt and black pepper to the taste
- A pinch of sweet paprika
- 1 tablespoon parsley, chopped
- 1 tablespoon lemon juice
- 1 tablespoon olive oil

Directions:

1. Season catfish fillets with salt, pepper, paprika, drizzle oil, rub well, place in your air fryer's basket and cook at 400 degrees F for 20 minutes, flipping the fish after 10 minutes.

2. Divide fish on plates, drizzle lemon juice all over, sprinkle parsley and serve.

3. Enjoy!

Nutrition Values: calories 253, fat 6, fiber 12, carbs 26, protein 22

Cod Fillets with Fennel and Grapes Salad

Preparation time: 10 minutes

Cooking time: 15 minutes

Servings: 2

Ingredients:

- 2 black cod fillets, boneless
- 1 tablespoon olive oil
- Salt and black pepper to the taste
- 1 fennel bulb, thinly sliced
- 1 cup grapes, halved
- ½ cup pecans

Directions:

1. Drizzle half of the oil over fish fillets, season with salt and pepper, rub well, place fillets in your air fryer's basket, cook for 10 minutes at 400 degrees F and transfer to a plate.

2. In a bowl, mix pecans with grapes, fennel, the rest of the oil, salt and pepper, toss to coat, add to a pan that fits your air fryer and cook at 400 degrees F for 5 minutes.

3. Divide cod on plates, add fennel and grapes mix on the side and serve.

4. Enjoy!

Nutrition Values: calories 300, fat 4, fiber 2, carbs 32, protein 22

Tabasco Shrimp

Preparation time: 10 minutes

Cooking time: 10 minutes

Servings: 4

Ingredients:

- 1 pound shrimp, peeled and deveined
- 1 teaspoon red pepper flakes
- 2 tablespoon olive oil
- 1 teaspoon Tabasco sauce
- 2 tablespoons water
- 1 teaspoon oregano, dried
- Salt and black pepper to the taste
- ½ teaspoon parsley, dried
- ½ teaspoon smoked paprika

Directions:

1. In a bowl, mix oil with water, Tabasco sauce, pepper flakes, oregano, parsley, salt, pepper, paprika and shrimp and toss well to coat.

2. Transfer shrimp to your preheated air fryer at 370 degrees F and cook for 10 minutes shaking the fryer once.

3. Divide shrimp on plates and serve with a side salad.

4. Enjoy!

Nutrition Values: calories 200, fat 5, fiber 6, carbs 13, protein 8

Buttered Shrimp Skewers

Preparation time: 10 minutes

Cooking time: 6 minutes

Servings: 2

Ingredients:

- 8 shrimps, peeled and deveined
- 4 garlic cloves, minced
- Salt and black pepper to the taste
- 8 green bell pepper slices
- 1 tablespoon rosemary, chopped
- 1 tablespoon butter, melted

Directions:

1. In a bowl, mix shrimp with garlic, butter, salt, pepper, rosemary and bell pepper slices, toss to coat and leave aside for 10 minutes.

2. Arrange 2 shrimp and 2 bell pepper slices on a skewer and repeat with the rest of the shrimp and bell pepper pieces.

3. Place them all in your air fryer's basket and cook at 360 degrees F for 6 minutes.

4. Divide among plates and serve right away.

5. Enjoy!

Nutrition Values: calories 140, fat 1, fiber 12, carbs 15, protein 7

Asian Salmon

Preparation time: 1 hour

Cooking time: 15 minutes

Servings: 2

Ingredients:

- 2 medium salmon fillets
- 6 tablespoons light soy sauce
- 3 teaspoons mirin
- 1 teaspoon water
- 6 tablespoons honey

Directions:

1. In a bowl, mix soy sauce with honey, water and mirin, whisk well, add salmon, rub well and leave aside in the fridge for 1 hour.

2. Transfer salmon to your air fryer and cook at 360 degrees F for 15 minutes, flipping them after 7 minutes.

3. Meanwhile, put the soy marinade in a pan, heat up over medium heat, whisk well, cook for 2 minutes and take off heat.

4. Divide salmon on plates, drizzle marinade all over and serve.

5. Enjoy!

Nutrition Values: calories 300, fat 12, fiber 8, carbs 13, protein 24

Cod Steaks with Plum Sauce

Preparation time: 10 minutes

Cooking time: 20 minutes

Servings: 2

Ingredients:

- 2 big cod steaks
- Salt and black pepper to the taste
- ½ teaspoon garlic powder
- ½ teaspoon ginger powder
- ¼ teaspoon turmeric powder
- 1 tablespoon plum sauce
- Cooking spray

Directions:

1. Season cod steaks with salt and pepper, spray them with cooking oil, add garlic powder, ginger powder and turmeric powder and rub well.

2. Place cod steaks in your air fryer and cook at 360 degrees F for 15 minutes, flipping them after 7 minutes.

3. Heat up a pan over medium heat, add plum sauce, stir and cook for 2 minutes.

4. Divide cod steaks on plates, drizzle plum sauce all over and serve.

5. Enjoy!

Nutrition Values: calories 250, fat 7, fiber 1, carbs 14, protein 12

Flavored Air Fried Salmon

Preparation time: 1 hour

Cooking time: 8 minutes

Servings: 2

Ingredients:

- 2 salmon fillets
- 2 tablespoons lemon juice
- Salt and black pepper to the taste
- ½ teaspoon garlic powder
- 1/3 cup water
- 1/3 cup soy sauce
- 3 scallions, chopped
- 1/3 cup brown sugar
- 2 tablespoons olive oil

Directions:

1. In a bowl, mix sugar with water, soy sauce, garlic powder, salt, pepper, oil and lemon juice, whisk well, add salmon fillets, toss to coat and leave aside in the fridge for 1 hour.

2. Transfer salmon fillets to the fryer's basket and cook at 360 degrees F for 8 minutes flipping them halfway.

3. Divide salmon on plates, sprinkle scallions on top and serve right away.

4. Enjoy!

Nutrition Values: calories 300, fat 12, fiber 10, carbs 23, protein 20

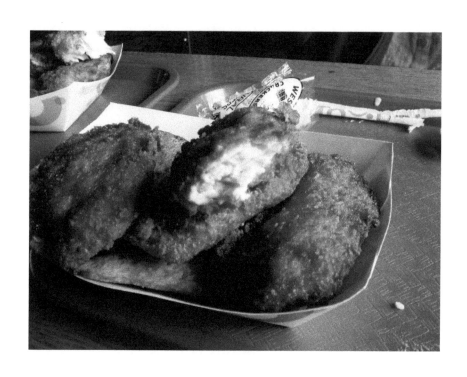

Salmon with Capers and Mash

Preparation time: 10 minutes

Cooking time: 20 minutes

Servings: 4

Ingredients:

- 4 salmon fillets, skinless and boneless
- 1 tablespoon capers, drained
- Salt and black pepper to the taste
- Juice from 1 lemon
- 2 teaspoons olive oil
- For the potato mash:
- 2 tablespoons olive oil
- 1 tablespoon dill, dried
- 1 pound potatoes, chopped
- ½ cup milk

Directions:

1. Put potatoes in a pot, add water to cover, add some salt, bring to a boil over medium high heat, cook for 15 minutes, drain, transfer to a bowl, mash with a potato masher, add 2 tablespoons oil, dill, salt, pepper and milk, whisk well and leave aside for now.

2. Season salmon with salt and pepper, drizzle 2 teaspoons oil over them, rub, transfer to your air fryer's basket, add capers on top, cook at 360 degrees F and cook for 8 minutes.

3. Divide salmon and capers on plates, add mashed potatoes on the side, drizzle lemon juice all over and serve.

4. Enjoy!

Nutrition Values: calories 300, fat 17, fiber 8, carbs 12, protein 18

Lemony Saba Fish

Preparation time: 10 minutes

Cooking time: 8 minutes

Servings: 1

Ingredients:

- 4 Saba fish fillet, boneless
- Salt and black pepper to the taste
- 3 red chili pepper, chopped
- 2 tablespoons lemon juice
- 2 tablespoon olive oil
- 2 tablespoon garlic, minced

Directions:

1. Season fish fillets with salt and pepper and put in a bowl.

2. Add lemon juice, oil, chili and garlic toss to coat, transfer fish to your air fryer and cook at 360 degrees F for 8 minutes, flipping halfway.

3. Divide among plates and serve with some fries.

4. Enjoy!

Nutrition Values: calories 300, fat 4, fiber 8, carbs 15, protein 15

Hash Brown Toasts

Preparation Time: 17 Minutes

Servings: 4

Ingredients:

- 4 hash brown patties; frozen
- 1 tbsp. olive oil
- 1 tbsp. balsamic vinegar
- 1 tbsp. basil; chopped.
- 1/4 cup cherry tomatoes; chopped.
- 3 tbsp. mozzarella; shredded
- 2 tbsp. parmesan; grated

Directions:

1. Put hash brown patties in your air fryer; drizzle the oil over them and cook them at 400 °F, for 7 minutes.

2. In a bowl; mix tomatoes with mozzarella, parmesan, vinegar and basil and stir well. Divide hash brown patties on plates; top each with tomatoes mix and serve for lunch.

Nutrition Values: Calories: 199; Fat: 3; Fiber: 8; Carbs: 12; Protein: 4

Creamy Potatoes

Preparation time: 5 minutes

Cooking time: 20 minutes

Servings: 4

Ingredients:

- 2 gold potatoes, cut into medium pieces
- 1 tablespoon olive oil
- Salt and black pepper to taste
- 3 tablespoons sour cream

Directions:

1. In a baking dish that fits your air fryer, mix all the ingredients and toss.

2. Place the dish in the air fryer and cook at 370 degrees F for 20 minutes.

3. Divide between plates and serve as a side dish.

Nutrition Values: calories 201, fat 8, fiber 9, carbs 18, protein 5

Sweet Potato Side Salad

Preparation time: 5 minutes

Cooking time: 20 minutes

Servings: 2

Ingredients:

- 2 sweet potatoes, peeled and cut into wedges
- Salt and black pepper to taste
- 2 tablespoons avocado oil
- ½ teaspoon curry powder
- ¼ teaspoon coriander, ground
- 4 tablespoons mayonnaise
- ½ teaspoon cumin, ground
- A pinch of ginger powder
- A pinch of cinnamon powder

Directions:

1. In your air fryer's basket, mix the sweet potato wedges with salt, pepper, coriander, curry powder, and the oil; toss well.

2. Cook at 370 degrees F for 20 minutes, flipping them once.

3. Transfer the potatoes to a bowl, then add the mayonnaise, cumin, ginger and the cinnamon.

4. Toss and serve as a side salad.

Nutrition Values: calories 190, fat 5, fiber 8, carbs 14, protein 5

Mayo Brussels Sprouts

Preparation time: 5 minutes

Cooking time: 15 minutes

Servings: 4

Ingredients:

- 1 pound Brussels sprouts, trimmed and halved
- Salt and black pepper to taste
- 6 teaspoons olive oil
- ½ cup mayonnaise
- 2 tablespoons garlic, minced

Directions:

1. In your air fryer, mix the sprouts, salt, pepper, and oil; toss well.

2. Cook the sprouts at 390 degrees F for 15 minutes.

3. Transfer them to a bowl; then add the mayo and the garlic and toss.

4. Divide between plates and serve as a side dish.

Nutrition Values: calories 202, fat 6, fiber 8, carbs 12, protein 8

Green Beans and Shallots

Preparation time: 5 minutes

Cooking time: 25 minutes

Servings: 4

Ingredients:

- 1½ pounds green beans, trimmed
- Salt and black pepper to taste
- ½ pound shallots, chopped
- ¼ cup walnuts, chopped
- 2 tablespoons olive oil

Directions:

1. In your air fryer, mix all ingredients and toss.

2. Cook at 350 degrees F for 25 minutes.

3. Divide between plates and serve as a side dish.

Nutrition Values: calories 182, fat 3, fiber 6, carbs 11, protein 5

107. Italian Mushroom Mix

Preparation time: 5 minutes

Cooking time: 15 minutes

Servings: 4

Ingredients:

- 1 pound button mushrooms, halved
- 2 tablespoons parmesan cheese, grated
- 1 teaspoon Italian seasoning
- A pinch of salt and black pepper
- 3 tablespoons butter, melted

Directions:

1. In a pan that fits your air fryer, mix all the ingredients and toss.

2. Place the pan in the air fryer and cook at 360 degrees F for 15 minutes.

3. Divide the mix between plates and serve.

Nutrition Values: calories 194, fat 4, fiber 4, carbs 14, protein 7

Crispy Fried Pickle Spears

Preparation Time: 15 minutes

Servings 6

Nutrition Values: 58 Calories; 2g Fat; 6.8g Carbs; 3.2g Protein; 0.9g Sugars

Ingredients

- 1/3 cup milk
- 1 teaspoon garlic powder
- 2 medium-sized eggs
- 1 teaspoon fine sea salt
- 1/3 teaspoon chili powder
- 1/3 cup all-purpose flour
- 1/2 teaspoon shallot powder
- 2 jars sweet and sour pickle spears

Directions

1. Pat the pickle spears dry with a kitchen towel. Then, take two mixing bowls.

2. Whisk the egg and milk in a bowl. In another bowl, combine all dry ingredients.

3. Firstly, dip the pickle spears into the dry mix; then coat each pickle with the egg/milk mixture; dredge them in the flour mixture again for additional coating.

4. Air fry battered pickles for 15 minutes at 385 degrees. Enjoy!

Spicy Winter Squash Bites

Preparation Time: 23 minutes

Servings 8

Nutrition Values:113 Calories; 3g Fat; 22.6g Carbs; 1.6g Protein; 4.3g Sugars

Ingredients

- 2 teaspoons fresh mint leaves, chopped

- 1/3 cup brown sugar

- 1 ½ teaspoons red pepper chili flakes

- 2 tablespoons melted butter

- 3 pounds winter squash, peeled, seeded, and cubed

Directions

1. Toss all of the above ingredients in a large-sized mixing dish.

2. Roast the squash bites for 30 minutes at 325 degrees F in your Air Fryer, turning once or twice. Serve with a homemade dipping sauce.

Butter Squash Fritters

Preparation Time: 22 minutes

Servings 4

Nutrition Values: 152 Calories; 10.02g Fat; 9.4g Carbs; 5.8g Protein; 0.3g Sugars

Ingredients

- 1/3 cup all-purpose flour
- 1/3 teaspoon freshly ground black pepper, or more to taste
- 1/3 teaspoon dried sage
- 4 cloves garlic, minced
- 1 ½ tablespoons olive oil
- 1/3 butternut squash, peeled and grated
- 2 eggs, well whisked
- 1 teaspoon fine sea salt
- A pinch of ground allspice

Directions

1. Thoroughly combine all ingredients in a mixing bowl.

2. Preheat your air fryer to 345 degrees and set the timer for 17 minutes; cook until your fritters are browned; serve right away.

Herbed Roasted Potatoes

Preparation Time: 24 minutes

Servings 4

Nutrition Values: 208 Calories; 7.1g Fat; 33.8g Carbs; 3.6g Protein; 2.5g Sugars

Ingredients

- 1 teaspoon crushed dried thyme
- 1 teaspoon ground black pepper
- 2 tablespoons olive oil
- 1/2 tablespoon crushed dried rosemary
- 3 potatoes, peeled, washed and cut into wedges
- 1/2 teaspoon seasoned salt

Directions

1. Lay the potatoes in the air fryer cooking basket; drizzle olive oil over your potatoes.

2. Then, cook for 17 minutes at 353 degrees F.

3. Toss with the seasonings and serve warm with your favorite salad on the side.

Indian-Style Garnet Sweet Potatoes

Preparation Time: 24 minutes

Servings 4

Nutrition Values: 103 Calories; 9.1g Fat; 4.9g Carbs; 1.9g Protein; 1.2g Sugars

Ingredients

- 1/3 teaspoon white pepper
- 1 tablespoon butter, melted
- 1/2 teaspoon turmeric powder
- 5 garnet sweet potatoes, peeled and diced
- 1 ½ tablespoons maple syrup
- 2 teaspoons tamarind paste
- 1 1/2 tablespoons fresh lime juice
- 1 1/2 teaspoon ground allspice

Directions

1. In a mixing bowl, toss all ingredients until sweet potatoes are well coated.

2. Air-fry them at 335 degrees F for 12 minutes.

3. Pause the air fryer and toss again. Increase the temperature to 390 degrees F and cook for an additional 10 minutes. Eat warm.

Easy Frizzled Leeks

Preparation Time: 52 minutes

Servings 6

> Nutrition Values:291 Calories; 6g Fat; 53.3g
> Carbs; 5.7g Protein; 4.3g Sugars

Ingredients

- 1/2 teaspoon porcini powder

- 1 1/2 cup rice flour

- 1 tablespoon vegetable oil

- 3 medium-sized leeks, slice into julienne strips

- 2 large-sized dishes with ice water

- 2 teaspoons onion powder

- Fine sea salt and cayenne pepper, to taste

Directions

1. Allow the leeks to soak in ice water for about 25 minutes; drain well.

2. Place the rice flour, salt, cayenne pepper, onions powder, and porcini powder into a

resealable bag. Add the celery and shake to coat well.

3. Drizzle vegetable oil over the seasoned leeks. Air fry at 390 degrees F for about 18 minutes; turn them halfway through the cooking time. Serve with homemade mayonnaise or any other sauce for dipping. Enjoy!

Cremini Mushrooms in Zesty Tahini Sauce

Preparation Time: 22 minutes

Servings 5

Nutrition Values: 372 Calories; 4g Fat; 80g Carbs; 11.2g Protein; 2.6g Sugars

Ingredients

- 1/2 tablespoon tahini
- 1/2 teaspoon turmeric powder
- 1/3 teaspoon cayenne pepper
- 2 tablespoons lemon juice, freshly squeezed
- 1 teaspoon kosher salt
- 1/3 teaspoon freshly cracked black pepper
- 1 1/2 tablespoons vermouth
- 1 ½ tablespoons olive oil
- 1 ½ pound Cremini mushrooms

Directions

1. Grab a mixing dish and toss the mushrooms with the olive oil, turmeric powder, salt, black pepper, and cayenne pepper.

2. Cook them in your air fryer for 9 minutes at 355 degrees F.

3. Pause your air fryer, give it a good stir and cook for 10 minutes longer.

4. Meanwhile, thoroughly combine lemon juice, vermouth, and tahini. Serve warm mushrooms with tahini sauce.

Hash Brown Casserole

Preparation Time: 23 minutes

Servings 6

Nutrition Values: 195 Calories; 11.1g Fat; 22g Carbs; 3.1g Protein; 3g Sugars

Ingredients

- 1/2 cup Cheddar cheese, shredded
- 1 tablespoon soft cheese, at room temperature
- 1/3 cup crushed bran cereal
- 1 ½ yellow or white medium-sized onion, chopped
- 5 ounces condensed cream of celery soup
- 1 tablespoons fresh cilantro, finely minced
- 1/3 cup sour cream
- 3 cloves garlic, peeled and finely minced
- 2 cups hash brown potatoes, shredded
- 1 1/2 tablespoons margarine or butter, melted

- Sea salt and freshly ground black pepper, to your liking

- Crushed red pepper flakes, to your liking

Directions

1. Grab a large-sized bowl and whisk the celery soup, sour cream, soft cheese, red pepper, salt, and black pepper. Stir in the hash browns, onion, garlic, cilantro, and Cheddar cheese. Mix until everything is thoroughly combined.

2. Scrape the mixture into a baking dish that is previously lightly greased.

3. In another mixing bowl, combine together the bran cereal and melted margarine -or butter. Spread the mixture evenly over the top of the hash brown mixture.

4. Bake for 17 minutes at 290 degrees F. Eat warm, garnished with some extra sour cream if desired.

Pepper Jack Cauliflower Bites

Preparation Time: 24 minutes

Servings 2

Nutrition Values: 271 Calories; 23g Fat; 8.9g Carbs; 9.8g Protein; 2.8g Sugars

Ingredients

- 1/3 teaspoon shallot powder
- 1 teaspoon ground black pepper
- 1 ½ large-sized heads of cauliflower, broken into florets
- 1/4 teaspoon cumin powder
- ½ teaspoon garlic salt
- 1/4 cup Pepper Jack cheese, grated
- 1 ½ tablespoons vegetable oil
- 1/3 teaspoon paprika

Directions

1. Boil cauliflower in a large pan of salted water approximately 5 minutes. After that,

drain the cauliflower florets; now, transfer them to a baking dish.

2. Toss the cauliflower florets with the rest of the above ingredients.

3. Roast at 395 degrees F for 16 minutes, turn them halfway through the process. Enjoy!

Cheesy Broccoli Croquettes

Preparation Time: 50 minutes

Servings 6

Nutrition Values: 246 Calories; 14g Fat; 15.2g Carbs; 14.5g Protein; 1.6g Sugars

Ingredients

- 1 1/2 cups Monterey Jack cheese
- 1 teaspoon dried dill weed
- 1/3 teaspoon ground black pepper
- 3 eggs, whisked
- 1 teaspoon cayenne pepper
- 1/2 teaspoon kosher salt
- 1 cup Panko crumbs
- 2 ½ cups broccoli florets
- 1/3 cup Parmesan cheese

Directions

1. Blitz the broccoli florets in a food processor until finely crumbed. Then, combine the

broccoli with the rest of the above ingredients.

2. Roll the mixture into small balls; place the balls in the fridge for approximately half an hour.

3. Preheat your air fryer to 335 degrees F and set the timer to 14 minutes; cook until broccoli croquettes are browned and serve warm.

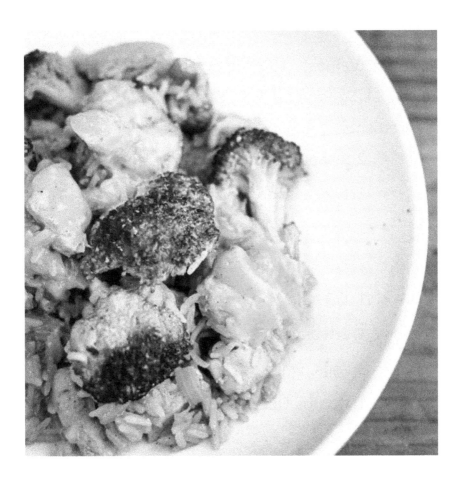

Cauliflower Cakes Ole

Preparation Time: 48 minutes

Servings 6

Nutrition Values: 190 Calories; 14.1g Fat; 4.7g Carbs; 11.5g Protein; 1.3g Sugars

Ingredients

- 2 teaspoons chili powder
- 1 1/2 teaspoon kosher salt
- 1 teaspoon dried marjoram, crushed
- 2 1/2 cups cauliflower, broken into florets
- 1 1/3 cups tortilla chip crumbs
- 1/2 teaspoon crushed red pepper flakes
- 3 eggs, whisked
- 1 ½ cups Queso cotija cheese, crumbled

Directions

1. Blitz the cauliflower florets in your food processor until they're crumbled -it is the size of rice. Then, combine the cauliflower "rice" with the other items.

2. Now, roll the cauliflower mixture into small balls; refrigerate for 30 minutes.

3. Preheat your air fryer to 345 degrees and set the timer for 14 minutes; cook until the balls are browned and serve right away.

Celery and Carrot Croquettes

Preparation Time: 25 minutes

Servings 4

Nutrition Values: 142 Calories; 6g Fat; 15.8g Carbs; 7.2g Protein; 3g Sugar s

Ingredients

- 2 small eggs, lightly beaten
- 1/3 teaspoon freshly cracked black pepper
- 1/3 cup Colby cheese, grated
- 1/2 tablespoon fresh dill, finely chopped
- 1/2 tablespoon garlic paste
- 1/3 cup onion, finely chopped
- 1/3 cup all-purpose flour
- 3 medium-sized carrots, trimmed and grated
- 2 teaspoons fine sea salt
- 3 medium-sized celery stalks, trimmed and grated

- 1/3 teaspoon baking powder

Directions

1. Place the carrots and celery on a paper towel and squeeze them to remove the excess liquid.

2. Combine the vegetables with the other ingredients in the order listed above. Shape the balls using 1 tablespoon of the vegetable mixture.

3. Then, gently flatten each ball with your palm or a wide spatula. Spritz the croquettes with a nonstick cooking oil.

4. Bake the vegetable cakes in a single layer for 17 minutes at 318 degrees F. Serve warm with sour cream.

Smoked Veggie Omelet

Preparation Time: 14 minutes

Servings 2

Nutrition Values: 226 Calories; 11.5g Fat; 14.2g Carbs; 16.3g Protein; 5.2g Sugars

Ingredients

- 1/3 cup cherry tomatoes, chopped
- 1 bell pepper, seeded and chopped
- 1/3 teaspoon freshly ground black pepper
- 1/2 purple onion, peeled and sliced
- 1 teaspoon smoked cayenne pepper
- 5 medium-sized eggs, well-beaten
- 1/3 cup smoked tofu, crumbled
- 1 teaspoon seasoned salt
- 1 1/2 tablespoons fresh chives, chopped

Directions

1. Brush a baking dish with a spray coating.

2. Throw all ingredients, minus fresh chives, into the baking dish; give it a good stir.

3. Cook about 15 minutes at 325 degrees F. Garnish with fresh chopped chives. Bon appétit!

Sweet Potato and Carrot Croquettes

Preparation Time: 22 minutes

Servings 4

Nutrition Values: 206 Calories; 5g Fat; 32g Carbs; 8.3g Protein; 5.7g Sugars

Ingredients

- 1/3 cup Swiss cheese, grated
- 1/3 teaspoon fine sea salt
- 1/3 teaspoon baking powder
- 1/3 cup scallions, finely chopped
- 1/2 tablespoon fresh basil, finely chopped
- 3 carrots, trimmed and grated
- 1/2 teaspoon freshly cracked black pepper
- 3 sweet potatoes, grated
- 1/3 cup all-purpose flour
- 2 small eggs, lightly beaten

Directions

1. Place grated sweet potatoes and carrots on a paper towel and pat them dry.

2. Combine the potatoes and carrots with the other ingredients in the order listed above. Then, create the balls using 1½ tablespoons of the vegetable mixture.

3. Then, gently flatten each ball. Spritz the croquettes with a nonstick cooking oil.

4. Bake your croquettes for 13 minutes at 305 degrees F; work with batches. Serve warm with tomato ketchup and mayonnaise.

Manchego and Potato Patties

Preparation Time: 15 minutes

Servings 8

Nutrition Values: 191 Calories; 8.7g Fat; 22g Carbs; 7g Protein; 1.4g Sugars

Ingredients

- 1 cup Manchego cheese, shredded
- 1 teaspoon paprika
- 1 teaspoon freshly ground black pepper
- 1/2 tablespoon fine sea salt
- 2 cups scallions, finely chopped
- 2 pounds Russet potatoes, peeled and grated
- 2 tablespoons canola oil
- 2 teaspoons dried basil

Directions

1. Thoroughly combine all of the above ingredients. Then, shape the balls using

your hands. Now, flatten the balls to make the patties.

2. Next, cook your patties at 360 degrees F approximately 10 minutes. Bon appétit!

Mint-Butter Stuffed Mushrooms

Preparation Time: 19 minutes

Servings 3

Nutrition Values:290 Calories; 14.7g Fat; 13.4g Carbs; 28g Protein; 3.3g Sugars

Ingredients

- 3 garlic cloves, minced
- 1 teaspoon ground black pepper, or more to taste
- 1/3 cup seasoned breadcrumbs
- 1½ tablespoons fresh mint, chopped
- 1 teaspoon salt, or more to taste
- 1½ tablespoons melted butter
- 14 medium-sized mushrooms, cleaned, stalks removed

Directions

1. Mix all of the above ingredients, minus the mushrooms, in a mixing bowl to prepare the filling.

2. Then, stuff the mushrooms with the prepared filling.

3. Air-fry stuffed mushrooms at 375 degrees F for about 12 minutes. Taste for doneness and serve at room temperature as a vegetarian appetizer.

Ricotta and Leafy Green Omelet

Preparation Time: 17 minutes

Servings 2

Nutrition Values: 409 Calories; 29.5g Fat; 6.9g Carbs; 27.9g Protein; 3g Sugars

Ingredients

- 1/3 cup Ricotta cheese
- 5 eggs, beaten
- 1/2 red bell pepper, seeded and sliced
- 1 cup mixed greens, roughly chopped
- 1/2 green bell pepper, seeded and sliced
- 1/2 teaspoon dried basil
- 1/2 chipotle pepper, finely minced
- 1/2 teaspoon dried oregano

Directions

1. Lightly coat the inside of a baking dish with a pan spray.

2. Then, throw all ingredients into the baking dish; give it a good stir.

3. Bake at 325 degrees F for 15 minutes.

Basic Pepper French Fries

Preparation Time: 33 minutes

Servings 4

Nutrition Values: 262 Calories; 9.1g Fat; 42g Carbs; 4.5g Protein; 3g Sugars

Ingredients

- 1 teaspoon fine sea salt

- 1/2 teaspoon freshly ground black pepper

- 2 ½ tablespoons canola oil

- 6 Russet potatoes, cut them into fries

- 1/2 teaspoon crushed red pepper flakes

Directions

1. Start by preheating your air fryer to 340 degrees F.

2. Place the fries in your air fryer and toss them with the oil. Add the seasonings and toss again.

3. Cook for 30 minutes, shaking your fries several times. Taste for doneness and eat warm.

Oyster Mushroom and Lemongrass Omelet

Preparation Time: 42 minutes

Servings 2

Nutrition Values: 362 Calories; 29g Fat; 7.2g Carbs; 19g Protein; 2.8g Sugars

Ingredients

- 3 king oyster mushrooms, thinly sliced
- 1 lemongrass, chopped
- 1/2 teaspoon dried marjoram
- 5 eggs
- 1/3 cup Swiss cheese, grated
- 2 tablespoons sour cream
- 1 1/2 teaspoon dried rosemary
- 2 teaspoons red pepper flakes, crushed
- 2 tablespoons butter, melted
- 1/2 red onion, peeled and sliced into thin rounds
- ½ teaspoon garlic powder

- 1 teaspoon dried dill weed
- Fine sea salt and ground black pepper, to your liking

Directions

1. Melt the margarine in a skillet that is placed over a medium flame. Then, sweat the onion, mushrooms, and lemongrass until they have softened; reserve.

2. Then, preheat the air fryer to 325 degrees F. Then, crack the eggs into a mixing bowl and whisk them well. Then, fold in the sour cream and give it a good stir.

3. Now, stir in the salt, black pepper, red pepper, rosemary, garlic powder, marjoram, and dill.

4. Next step, grease the inside of an air fryer baking dish with a thin layer of a cooking spray. Pour the egg/seasoning mixture into the baking dish; throw in the reserved mixture. Top with the Swiss cheese.

5. Set the timer for 35 minutes; cook until a knife inserted in the center comes out clean and dry

Spinach and Cheese Stuffed Baked Potatoes

Preparation Time: 18 minutes

Servings 4

Nutrition Values: 327 Calories; 7g Fat; 59g Carbs; 9.4g Protein; 2.2g Sugars

Ingredients

- 3 tablespoons extra-virgin olive oil
- 2/3 cup sour cream, at room temperature
- 1½ cup baby spinach leaves, torn into small pieces
- 3 pounds russet potatoes
- 2 garlic cloves, peeled and finely minced
- 1/4 teaspoon fine sea salt, or more to taste
- 1/4 teaspoon freshly cracked black pepper, or more to taste
- 1/3 cup Cheddar cheese, freshly grated

Directions

1. Firstly, stab the potatoes with a fork. Preheat the air fryer to 345 degrees F. Now, cook the potatoes for 14 minutes.

2. Meanwhile, make the filling by mixing the rest of the above items.

3. Afterward that, open the potatoes up and stuff them with the prepared filling. Bon appétit!

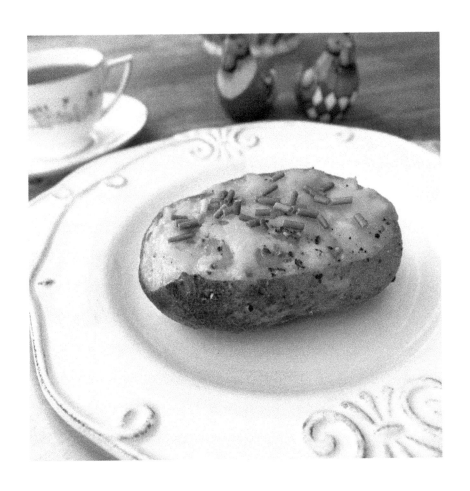

Lightning Source UK Ltd.
Milton Keynes UK
UKHW020640220621
385951UK00004B/91